This publication is intended to provide educational information for the reader on the covered subjects. It is not intended to take the place of personalized medical counseling, diagnosis, and treatment from a trained healthcare professional.

ISBN 978-1-998381-77-7 (Paperback)
ISBN 978-1-998381-78-4 (eBook)

Printed and bound in USA
Published by Loons Press

LOONS PRESS

Table Of Contents

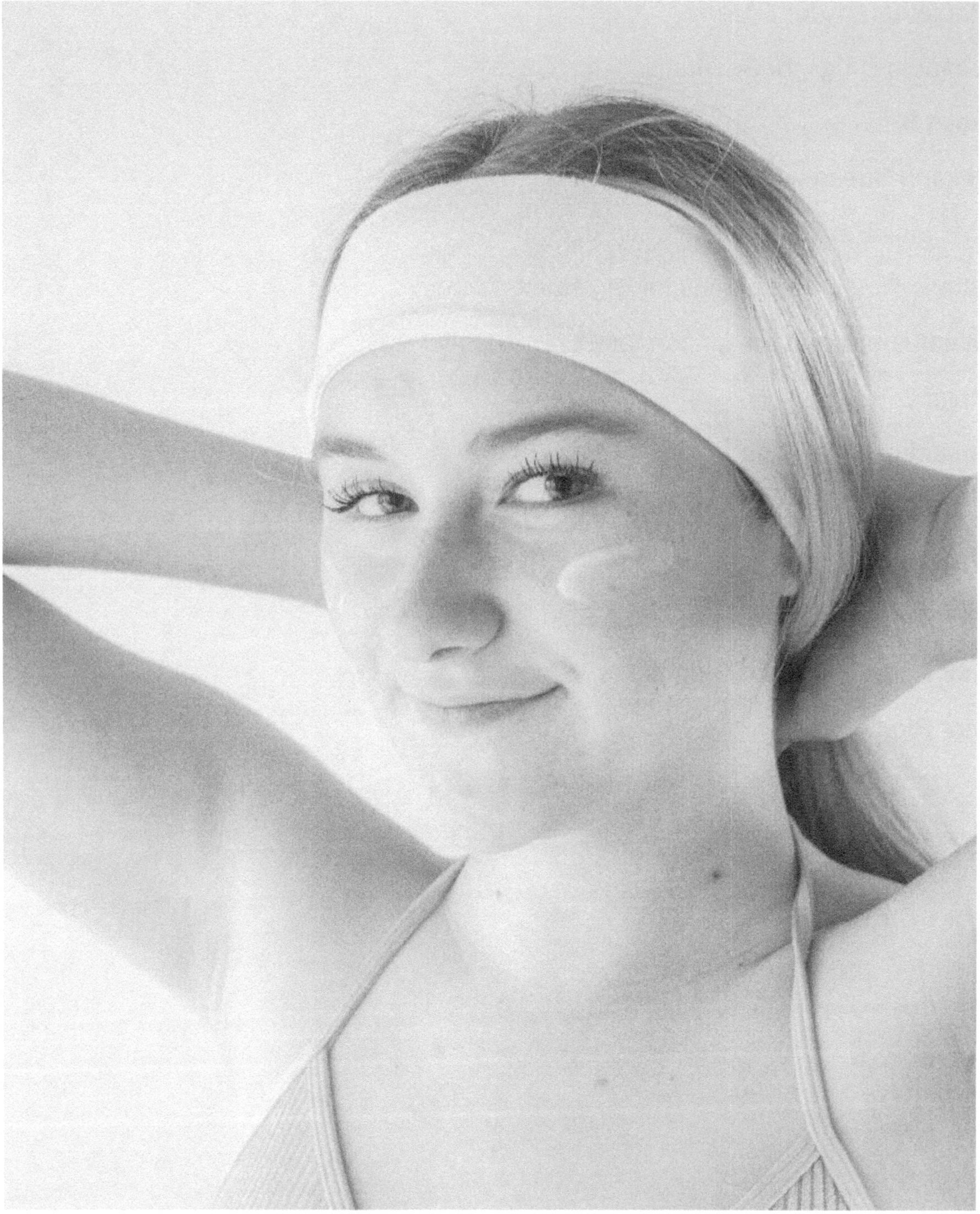

Chapter 1

Understanding Eczema

What is Eczema?

Eczema is a common skin condition that affects millions of people worldwide. It is characterized by red, inflamed, and itchy patches of skin that can be both uncomfortable and unsightly. Eczema can occur on any part of the body, but it is most commonly found on the hands, arms, face, and legs.

One of the key features of eczema is its chronic nature, meaning that it can flare up repeatedly over time. This can be frustrating for those who suffer from the condition, as it can be difficult to manage and control. Eczema is often triggered by a combination of genetic and environmental factors, such as stress, allergies, and irritants in the environment.

There are several different types of eczema, including atopic dermatitis, contact dermatitis, and nummular eczema. Each type has its own set of symptoms and triggers, but they all share the common characteristic of causing red, itchy skin.

Fortunately, there are many ways to manage and treat eczema. This can include using moisturizers to keep the skin hydrated, avoiding triggers such as harsh soaps and detergents, and using topical corticosteroids to reduce inflammation. In severe cases, oral medications or light therapy may be necessary.

By understanding the nature of eczema and learning how to properly care for your skin, you can take control of your condition and improve your quality of life. With the right knowledge and treatment plan, you can effectively manage your eczema and enjoy clear, healthy skin once again.

Causes of Eczema

Eczema is a common skin condition that affects millions of people worldwide. While the exact cause of eczema is still unknown, there are several factors that are believed to contribute to the development of this condition.

One of the main causes of eczema is genetics. If you have a family history of eczema, you are more likely to develop the condition yourself. This is because certain genes can make you more susceptible to developing eczema.

Another common cause of eczema is a weakened immune system. When your immune system is not functioning properly, it can overreact to certain triggers, such as allergens or irritants, leading to inflammation and irritation of the skin.

Environmental factors can also play a role in the development of eczema. Exposure to harsh chemicals, extreme temperatures, or dry air can all trigger eczema flare-ups in susceptible individuals.

Stress is another major cause of eczema. When you are stressed, your body releases certain hormones that can exacerbate inflammation in the skin, leading to flare-ups of eczema.

Lastly, certain foods and allergens can also trigger eczema in some individuals. Common food triggers for eczema include dairy, eggs, nuts, and gluten. Identifying and avoiding these triggers can help to prevent flare-ups of eczema.

By understanding the potential causes of eczema, you can take steps to avoid triggers and manage your condition more effectively. From addressing genetic predispositions to managing stress levels and avoiding allergens, there are many ways to help heal eczema and achieve clearer, healthier skin.

Types of Eczema

Eczema is a common skin condition that affects millions of people around the world. There are several different types of eczema, each with its own unique characteristics and triggers. Understanding the different types of eczema is essential for effectively managing and treating the condition.

One of the most common types of eczema is atopic dermatitis, which is characterized by dry, itchy, and inflamed skin. This type of eczema is often genetic and can be triggered by environmental factors such as allergens and irritants. Contact dermatitis is another common type of eczema, which occurs when the skin comes into contact with a substance that causes an allergic reaction.

Other types of eczema include nummular eczema, which causes coin-shaped patches of irritated skin, and dyshidrotic eczema, which results in blisters on the hands and feet. Seborrheic dermatitis is a type of eczema that primarily affects the scalp and face, causing redness, flaking, and itching.

Understanding the specific type of eczema you have is crucial for developing an effective treatment plan. By identifying your triggers and avoiding them, you can help prevent flare-ups and manage your symptoms more effectively. Working with a dermatologist or healthcare provider can help you determine the best course of action for your specific type of eczema.

In "Eczema-Free: The Ultimate Guide to Clearing Up Your Skin," we delve into the different types of eczema and provide practical tips and strategies for managing each type. By arming yourself with knowledge and understanding, you can take control of your eczema and work towards achieving clear, healthy skin.

Common Triggers for Eczema Flare-ups

Eczema, also known as atopic dermatitis, is a chronic skin condition that can be triggered by a variety of factors. Understanding these triggers is crucial for managing and preventing flare-ups. In this chapter, we will explore some of the most common triggers for eczema flare-ups and provide tips on how to avoid them.

One of the primary triggers for eczema flare-ups is dry skin. When the skin becomes dry and dehydrated, it can become more prone to irritation and inflammation. To combat this, it is essential to moisturize regularly with a gentle, fragrance-free moisturizer.

Another common trigger for eczema flare-ups is exposure to certain allergens. These can include pet dander, dust mites, pollen, and certain foods. It is important to identify and avoid these triggers to prevent flare-ups. Allergy testing may be necessary to pinpoint specific allergens.

Stress is also a significant trigger for eczema flare-ups. When we are stressed, our bodies release hormones that can exacerbate inflammation in the skin. Finding healthy ways to manage stress, such as through exercise, meditation, or therapy, can help prevent flare-ups.

Other common triggers for eczema flare-ups include harsh soaps and detergents, extreme temperatures, and certain fabrics. Avoiding these triggers and opting for gentle, hypoallergenic products can help keep eczema at bay.

By being aware of these common triggers and taking steps to avoid them, you can help prevent eczema flare-ups and keep your skin clear and healthy. Remember, everyone's triggers may be different, so it may take some time and experimentation to figure out what works best for you. But with patience and persistence, you can find relief from eczema and enjoy healthy, clear skin once again.

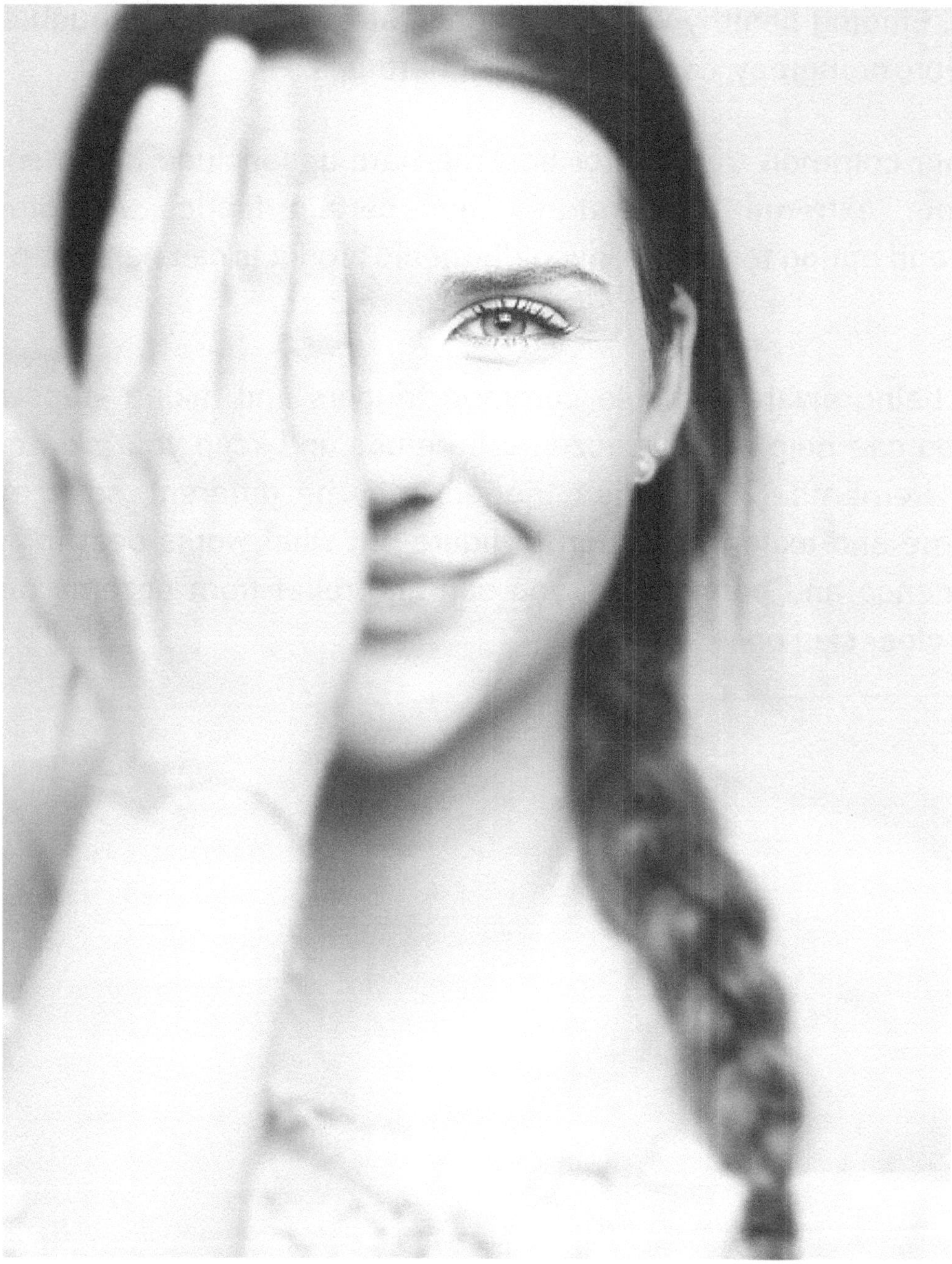

Chapter 2

Identifying Your Eczema Triggers

Keeping a Symptom Diary

Keeping a symptom diary is a crucial step in effectively managing and eventually healing eczema. By documenting your symptoms on a daily basis, you can identify patterns and triggers that may be exacerbating your condition. This valuable information can help you and your healthcare provider develop a personalized treatment plan that targets the root cause of your eczema.

To start your symptom diary, create a simple log where you can record details such as the date, time, location, and severity of your symptoms. Note any environmental factors that may have contributed to flare-ups, such as exposure to certain allergens or irritants. It's also important to document any changes in your skincare routine, diet, stress levels, or other lifestyle factors that could impact your skin health.

By consistently tracking your symptoms, you may begin to notice trends that can guide you in making informed decisions about your eczema management. For example, you may discover that certain foods or fabrics trigger your symptoms, or that stress and lack of sleep worsen your eczema flare-ups. Armed with this knowledge, you can take proactive steps to avoid these triggers and create a more eczema-friendly environment for your skin.

Remember to be patient and persistent in keeping your symptom diary. Healing eczema is a journey that requires dedication and a willingness to make lifestyle changes. By staying committed to tracking your symptoms and working closely with your healthcare provider, you can take control of your eczema and achieve clearer, healthier skin.

Common Eczema Triggers to Look Out For

Eczema is a common skin condition that affects millions of people worldwide. While the exact cause of eczema is still unknown, there are several common triggers that can exacerbate symptoms and lead to flare-ups. By identifying and avoiding these triggers, individuals can better manage their eczema and improve the overall health of their skin.

One of the most common triggers for eczema is dry skin. When the skin becomes dry and dehydrated, it is more prone to irritation and inflammation, which can worsen eczema symptoms. To combat dry skin, it is important to regularly moisturize with a gentle, fragrance-free moisturizer and avoid harsh soaps and detergents that can strip the skin of its natural oils.

Another common trigger for eczema is stress. Stress can weaken the immune system and increase inflammation in the body, making it more difficult for the skin to heal. To reduce stress levels, individuals can practice mindfulness techniques such as deep breathing, meditation, and yoga, as well as engage in regular exercise and maintain a healthy diet.

Certain foods can also trigger eczema flare-ups in some individuals. Common food triggers include dairy, gluten, nuts, and eggs. By keeping a food diary and tracking symptoms, individuals can identify which foods may be exacerbating their eczema and eliminate them from their diet.

Other common triggers for eczema include harsh weather conditions, allergens such as pet dander and pollen, and irritants such as fragrances and chemicals in skincare products. By identifying and avoiding these triggers, individuals can better manage their eczema and improve the overall health of their skin.

In conclusion, by being aware of common eczema triggers and taking proactive steps to avoid them, individuals can better manage their eczema and achieve clearer, healthier skin. By incorporating these tips into their daily routine, individuals can take control of their eczema and live a happier, healthier life.

How to Avoid Eczema Triggers

Eczema can be a frustrating and uncomfortable skin condition, but there are steps you can take to avoid triggers that may exacerbate your symptoms. By making simple changes to your lifestyle and environment, you can help reduce flare-ups and keep your skin clear and healthy.

One of the most important things you can do to avoid eczema triggers is to identify what causes your flare-ups. Keep a journal of your symptoms and note any patterns or correlations with certain foods, products, or environmental factors. This can help you pinpoint your triggers and make necessary adjustments to your routine.

Avoiding harsh chemicals and fragrances in your skincare products and household cleaners can also help prevent eczema flare-ups. Opt for gentle, fragrance-free products that are specifically designed for sensitive skin. Additionally, choose clothing made from soft, breathable fabrics like cotton and avoid wearing tight, irritating clothing that can rub against your skin.

Maintaining a healthy diet rich in fruits, vegetables, and whole grains can also help prevent eczema flare-ups. Some people find that certain foods like dairy, gluten, or nuts can trigger their symptoms, so it may be helpful to eliminate these foods from your diet and see if it makes a difference.

Finally, managing stress and getting enough sleep are crucial for maintaining healthy skin and preventing eczema flare-ups. Practice relaxation techniques like deep breathing, meditation, or yoga to reduce stress levels, and aim for at least 7-8 hours of quality sleep each night.

By taking proactive steps to avoid eczema triggers, you can help keep your skin clear and comfortable. Remember, everyone's triggers are different, so it may take some trial and error to find what works best for you. Stay patient and persistent, and don't be afraid to seek help from a dermatologist if you need additional support.

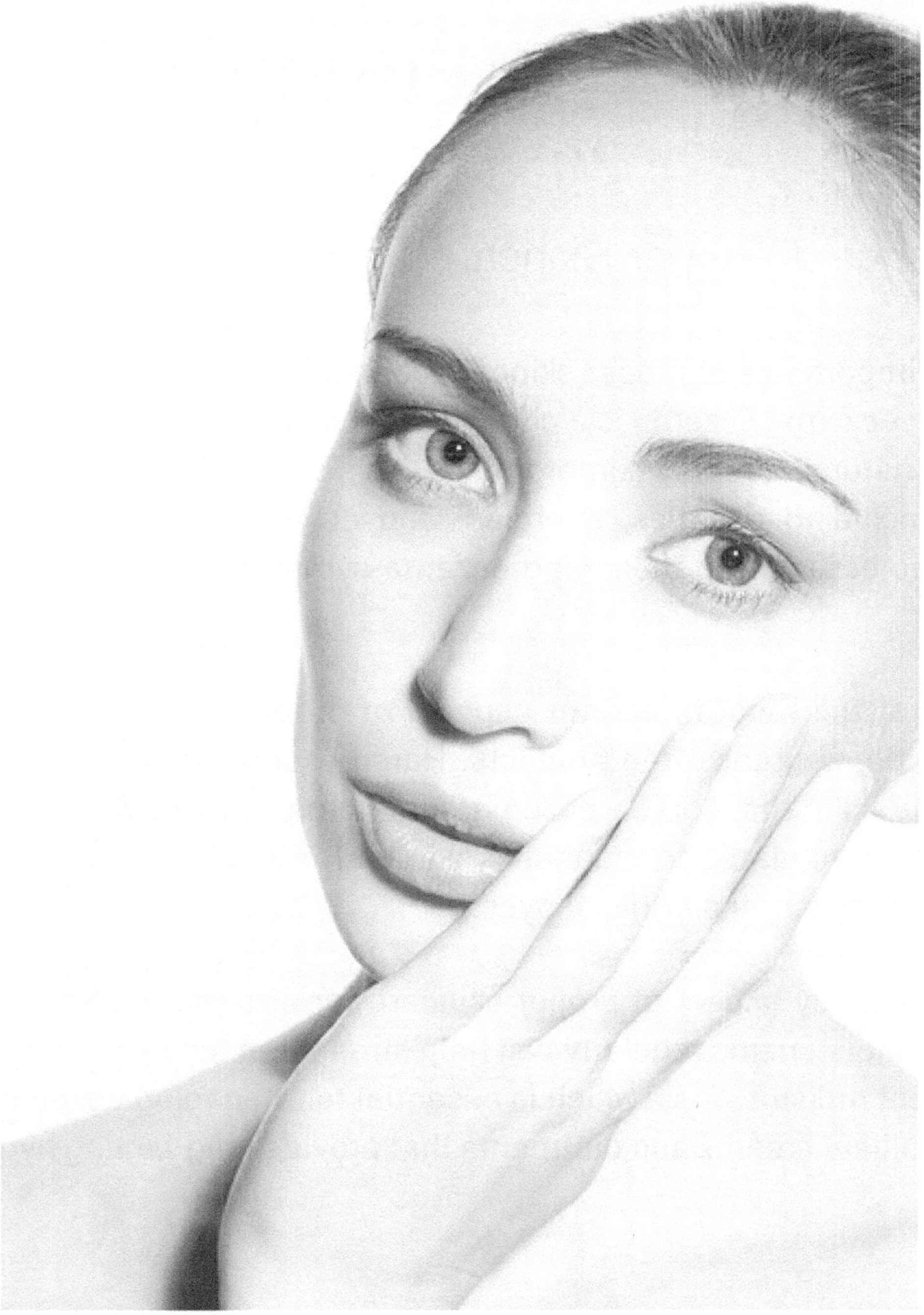

Chapter 3

Creating a Skin-Healthy Lifestyle

Importance of Proper Skincare

The importance of proper skincare cannot be overstated when it comes to healing eczema. Eczema is a chronic skin condition that can flare up when the skin's natural barrier is compromised. This can happen due to a variety of factors, including genetics, allergies, and environmental triggers. Proper skincare is essential in managing eczema symptoms and preventing flare-ups.

One of the most important aspects of proper skincare for eczema is using gentle, fragrance-free products. Harsh chemicals and fragrances can irritate the skin and worsen eczema symptoms. Opt for products that are specifically formulated for sensitive skin and free of common irritants like parabens, sulfates, and artificial dyes.

Another key aspect of proper skincare for eczema is keeping the skin hydrated. Moisturizing regularly can help strengthen the skin's natural barrier and prevent moisture loss, which is essential for managing eczema. Look for thick, emollient creams and ointments that provide long-lasting hydration.

In addition to using gentle products and keeping the skin well-hydrated, it's important to avoid common triggers that can aggravate eczema. These triggers can vary from person to person but may include things like certain foods, stress, and environmental factors like pollen or pet dander. Pay attention to your body and take note of any patterns or triggers that seem to worsen your eczema symptoms.

By following a proper skincare routine and being mindful of potential triggers, you can help manage your eczema symptoms and prevent flare-ups. Remember, healing eczema is a journey, and finding the right skincare routine that works for you may take some trial and error. Be patient with yourself and your skin, and don't hesitate to seek guidance from a dermatologist or skincare professional if needed.

Choosing the Right Products for Eczema-Prone Skin

When it comes to managing eczema-prone skin, choosing the right products is essential. With so many options on the market, it can be overwhelming to know where to start. However, by following some guidelines, you can select products that will help soothe and heal your skin.

First and foremost, look for products that are specifically designed for sensitive skin. These products are usually free of harsh chemicals, fragrances, and dyes that can exacerbate eczema symptoms. Opt for gentle cleansers, moisturizers, and other skincare products that are labeled as hypoallergenic and non-comedogenic.

Next, pay attention to the ingredients in the products you choose. Avoid products that contain common allergens such as parabens, sulfates, and artificial fragrances. Instead, look for ingredients like colloidal oatmeal, ceramides, and hyaluronic acid, which can help hydrate and protect the skin barrier.

It's also important to consider the texture of the products you use. For eczema-prone skin, lightweight, non-greasy formulas are usually best. Avoid heavy creams and ointments that can clog pores and worsen inflammation.

When selecting skincare products, it's a good idea to patch test them first. Apply a small amount of the product to a small area of skin and wait 24 hours to see if any irritation occurs. This can help you avoid potential flare-ups and reactions.

By choosing the right products for your eczema-prone skin, you can help alleviate symptoms and promote healing. Remember to consult with a dermatologist if you have any questions or concerns about which products are best for your specific skin type.

Dietary Changes for Eczema Relief

If you're looking for relief from eczema, making dietary changes can play a significant role in improving your skin condition. By incorporating certain foods and eliminating others, you can potentially see a reduction in eczema flare-ups and experience clearer, healthier skin.

One of the first steps in making dietary changes for eczema relief is to identify any potential trigger foods that may be exacerbating your symptoms. Common trigger foods for eczema include dairy, gluten, nuts, and eggs. Keeping a food diary can help you track your intake and identify any patterns between certain foods and flare-ups.

Incorporating anti-inflammatory foods into your diet can also help reduce inflammation associated with eczema. Foods rich in omega-3 fatty acids, such as salmon, flaxseeds, and walnuts, can help reduce inflammation and promote healthier skin. Additionally, foods high in antioxidants, such as berries, leafy greens, and turmeric, can help protect your skin from oxidative stress and improve overall skin health.

Hydration is key when it comes to managing eczema. Drinking plenty of water throughout the day can help keep your skin hydrated and reduce dryness and irritation. Limiting your intake of sugary and caffeinated beverages can also help prevent dehydration and support healthy skin.

In conclusion, making dietary changes for eczema relief can have a significant impact on your skin health. By identifying trigger foods, incorporating anti-inflammatory foods, and staying hydrated, you can take proactive steps towards healing your eczema and achieving clearer, healthier skin. Remember to consult with a healthcare professional or nutritionist before making any drastic changes to your diet.

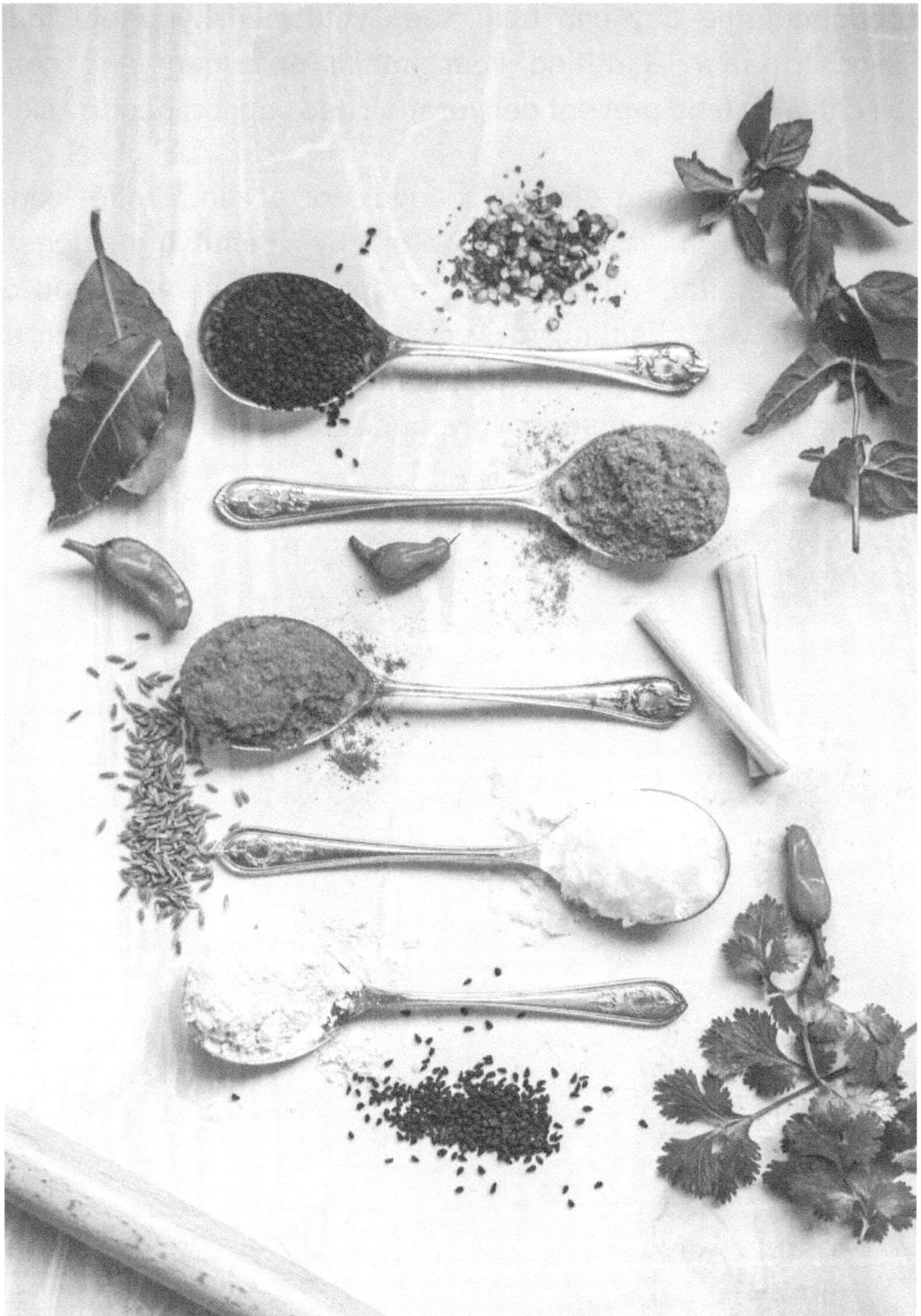

Chapter 4

Natural Remedies for Eczema

Soothing Baths and Moisturizers

One of the most effective ways to manage and heal eczema is through the use of soothing baths and moisturizers. Eczema, also known as atopic dermatitis, can cause dry, itchy, and inflamed skin that can be uncomfortable and even painful. By incorporating soothing baths and moisturizers into your skincare routine, you can help to alleviate these symptoms and promote healing for your skin.

When it comes to taking a soothing bath, there are a few key ingredients that can help to calm irritated skin and provide relief from itching. Adding colloidal oatmeal, baking soda, or Epsom salts to your bathwater can help to soothe inflamed skin and reduce itchiness. Additionally, using lukewarm water instead of hot water can help to prevent further irritation of your skin.

After your bath, it's important to moisturize your skin to lock in hydration and prevent dryness. Look for moisturizers that are gentle, fragrance-free, and specifically formulated for sensitive skin. Ingredients like ceramides, hyaluronic acid, and shea butter can help to repair the skin barrier and keep your skin hydrated and healthy.

Consistency is key when it comes to using soothing baths and moisturizers to heal eczema. Make sure to incorporate these treatments into your daily skincare routine to see the best results. By taking care of your skin with gentle, nourishing products, you can help to manage your eczema symptoms and achieve clear, healthy skin.

Herbal Supplements for Eczema

Eczema is a common skin condition that affects millions of people worldwide. While there is no cure for eczema, there are various treatments available to help manage and alleviate symptoms. One natural approach that many individuals have found to be effective in treating eczema is the use of herbal supplements.

Herbal supplements for eczema can offer a natural alternative to traditional medications and creams. These supplements are often derived from plants and herbs that have anti-inflammatory and soothing properties, making them ideal for calming irritated skin and reducing the redness and itchiness associated with eczema.

One popular herbal supplement for eczema is evening primrose oil, which is rich in gamma-linolenic acid (GLA). GLA is an essential fatty acid that has been shown to help reduce inflammation and improve skin hydration, making it an excellent choice for individuals with eczema.

Another herbal supplement that may be beneficial for eczema is turmeric. Turmeric contains curcumin, a compound that has powerful anti-inflammatory and antioxidant properties. Studies have shown that curcumin can help reduce inflammation in the skin and improve symptoms of eczema.

Other herbal supplements that may be beneficial for eczema include aloe vera, chamomile, and calendula. These herbs have been used for centuries for their healing properties and can help soothe and nourish the skin, making them a great addition to any eczema treatment regimen.

Before starting any herbal supplements for eczema, it is important to consult with a healthcare provider or dermatologist to ensure they are safe and appropriate for your individual needs. Additionally, it is essential to remember that herbal supplements are not a substitute for medical treatment and should be used in conjunction with other eczema management strategies, such as proper skincare, diet, and lifestyle changes.

In conclusion, herbal supplements can be a valuable addition to your eczema treatment plan. By incorporating these natural remedies into your daily routine, you may find relief from the symptoms of eczema and experience healthier, clearer skin.

Essential Oils for Eczema Relief

If you're struggling with eczema and looking for natural remedies to help soothe your skin, essential oils may be the answer you've been searching for. These powerful plant extracts have been used for centuries for their healing properties and can provide relief from the symptoms of eczema.

One of the most popular essential oils for eczema relief is lavender oil. Known for its calming and anti-inflammatory properties, lavender oil can help reduce redness, itching, and inflammation associated with eczema. Simply dilute a few drops of lavender oil with a carrier oil like coconut or almond oil and apply it to the affected areas of your skin for soothing relief.

Tea tree oil is another essential oil that can be beneficial for eczema sufferers. This powerful oil has antibacterial and anti-inflammatory properties that can help reduce itching and redness caused by eczema flare-ups. Mix a few drops of tea tree oil with a carrier oil and apply it to your skin to help alleviate symptoms and promote healing.

Chamomile oil is another great option for those looking to relieve eczema symptoms naturally. This gentle essential oil has anti-inflammatory and calming properties that can help soothe irritated skin and reduce itching. Mix chamomile oil with a carrier oil and apply it to your skin for relief from eczema discomfort.

When using essential oils for eczema relief, it's important to remember to always dilute them with a carrier oil to prevent irritation. Additionally, it's a good idea to do a patch test before using any new essential oil to ensure you don't have any adverse reactions.

Incorporating essential oils into your eczema treatment regimen can provide natural relief from symptoms and help promote healing. Experiment with different oils to find the ones that work best for your skin, and enjoy the soothing benefits of these powerful plant extracts on your journey to clearer, healthier skin.

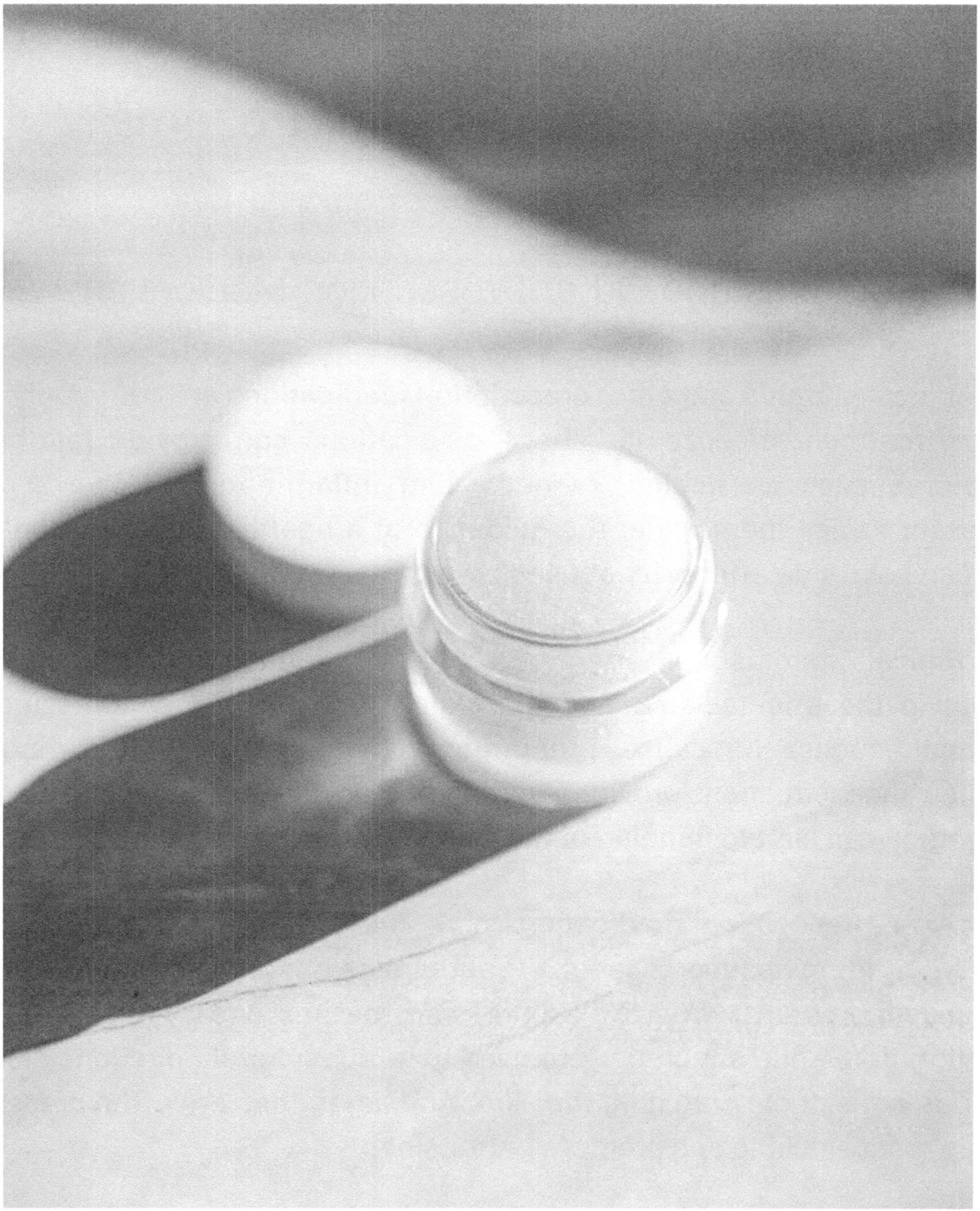

Chapter 5

Medical Treatments for Eczema

Topical Steroids and Other Prescription Medications

Topical steroids and other prescription medications are commonly used in the treatment of eczema. These medications can provide relief from symptoms such as itching, redness, and inflammation. However, it is important to use them under the guidance of a healthcare professional, as they can have side effects if not used correctly.

Topical steroids are often prescribed to reduce inflammation and itching in the affected areas of the skin. They work by suppressing the immune response that causes inflammation in the first place. It is important to follow the instructions provided by your doctor when using topical steroids, as overuse can lead to thinning of the skin and other side effects.

Other prescription medications that may be used to treat eczema include immunosuppressants, antibiotics, and antihistamines. Immunosuppressants work by suppressing the immune system to reduce inflammation, while antibiotics are used to treat bacterial infections that can occur as a result of scratching the skin. Antihistamines are often prescribed to help reduce itching and promote better sleep.

In addition to prescription medications, there are also non-prescription options available for treating eczema. These include over-the-counter corticosteroid creams, moisturizers, and antihistamine creams. It is important to discuss these options with your healthcare provider to determine the best treatment plan for your individual needs.

Overall, topical steroids and other prescription medications can be effective in treating eczema symptoms. However, it is important to use them as directed and to monitor for any potential side effects. With proper care and treatment, it is possible to manage and heal eczema effectively.

Phototherapy for Eczema

Phototherapy, also known as light therapy, is a non-invasive treatment option for individuals suffering from eczema. This form of therapy involves exposing the skin to ultraviolet (UV) light in a controlled environment to help reduce inflammation, itching, and redness associated with eczema.

There are different types of phototherapy available for eczema, including UVB (ultraviolet B) and UVA (ultraviolet A) therapy. UVB therapy is often used for treating mild to moderate eczema, while UVA therapy is typically reserved for more severe cases. Both types of phototherapy work by suppressing the immune system in the skin and reducing inflammation.

One of the main benefits of phototherapy for eczema is that it can be a safe and effective treatment option for individuals who may not respond well to traditional topical medications or oral treatments. Additionally, phototherapy can be used in conjunction with other treatments to help improve overall skin health and reduce flare-ups.

It is important to note that phototherapy should always be performed under the guidance of a healthcare professional, as overexposure to UV light can increase the risk of skin cancer. Your healthcare provider will determine the appropriate dosage and frequency of phototherapy sessions based on your individual needs and medical history.

Overall, phototherapy can be a valuable tool in managing eczema symptoms and improving the overall health of your skin. If you are considering phototherapy as a treatment option for eczema, be sure to consult with your healthcare provider to discuss the potential benefits and risks associated with this form of therapy.

Biologic Drugs for Severe Eczema Cases

For individuals suffering from severe cases of eczema, traditional treatments such as topical creams and oral medications may not always provide the relief they need. In these cases, biologic drugs may be recommended as a more effective treatment option.

Biologic drugs are a newer class of medications that target specific parts of the immune system involved in the inflammatory response seen in eczema. By targeting these specific pathways, biologic drugs can help reduce inflammation and improve symptoms in individuals with severe eczema.

One of the most commonly used biologic drugs for severe eczema is Dupilumab. This medication works by blocking the action of certain proteins in the body that contribute to the inflammation associated with eczema. Clinical trials have shown that Dupilumab can significantly improve symptoms, including reducing itchiness and redness, and promoting clearer skin in individuals with severe eczema.

It is important to note that biologic drugs are typically reserved for individuals with severe eczema that has not responded well to other treatments. These medications are usually given as injections or infusions and may have potential side effects, so it is important to work closely with a healthcare provider to determine if biologic drugs are the right treatment option for you.

Overall, biologic drugs offer a promising treatment option for individuals with severe eczema who have not found relief with other treatments. By targeting specific parts of the immune system, these medications can help improve symptoms and quality of life for those struggling with severe eczema.

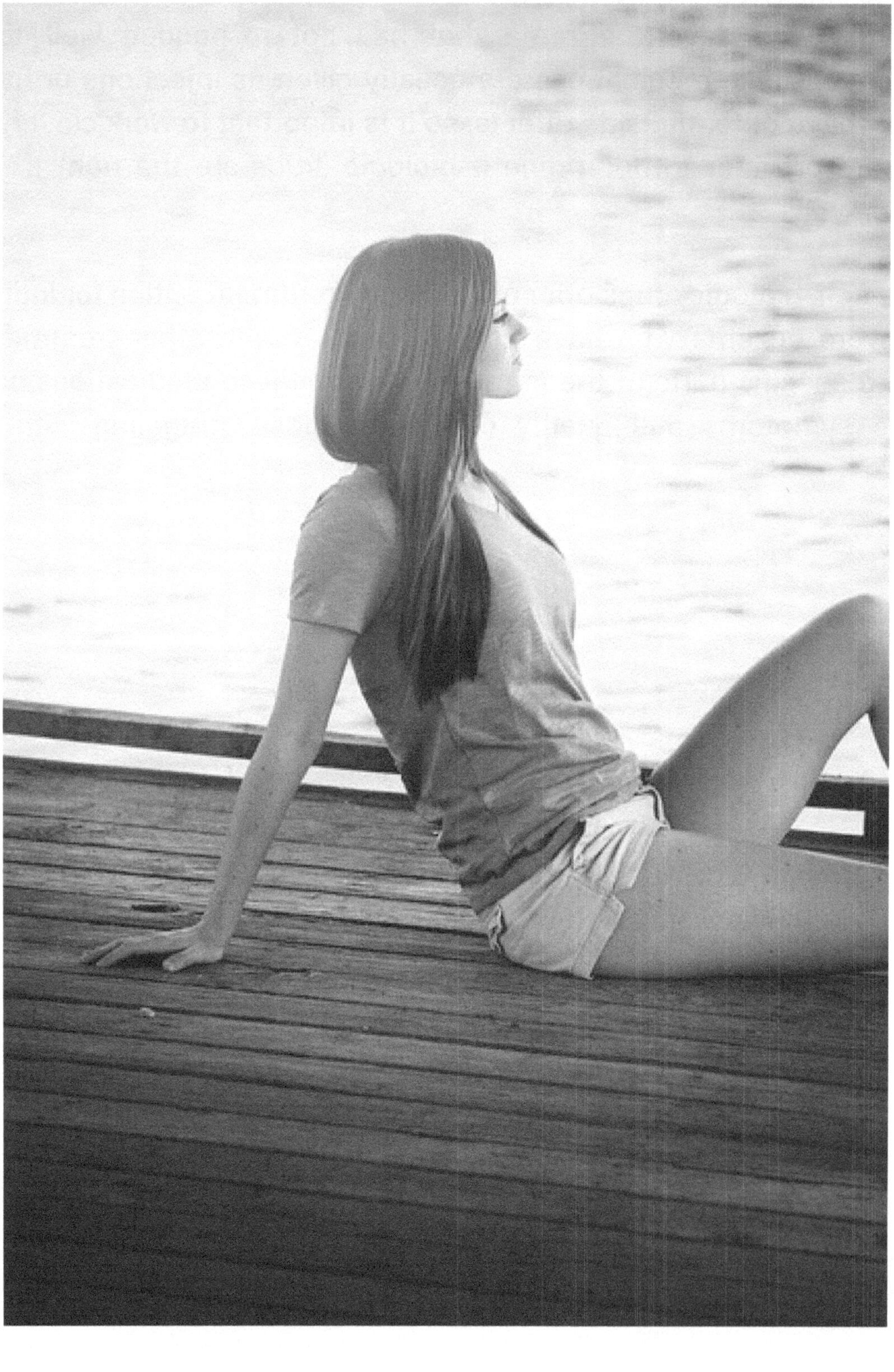

Chapter 6

Managing Stress and Eczema

The Link Between Stress and Eczema

Eczema is a common skin condition that affects millions of people worldwide. While the exact cause of eczema is not fully understood, there is evidence to suggest that stress can play a significant role in exacerbating symptoms. In this subchapter, we will explore the link between stress and eczema, and how managing stress can help improve the condition of your skin.

Stress is known to trigger the body's inflammatory response, which can worsen eczema symptoms such as redness, itching, and flaking. When we are stressed, our bodies release hormones like cortisol, which can lead to increased inflammation in the skin. This inflammation can cause the skin to become more irritated and sensitive, making eczema flare-ups more likely.

In addition to triggering inflammation, stress can also weaken the skin's natural barrier function, making it more susceptible to irritants and allergens that can exacerbate eczema symptoms. This can lead to a vicious cycle of stress causing eczema flare-ups, which in turn causes more stress, creating a feedback loop that can be difficult to break.

Fortunately, there are ways to manage stress and reduce its impact on your skin. Practices such as mindfulness meditation, deep breathing exercises, and yoga can help calm the mind and body, reducing cortisol levels and promoting relaxation. Regular exercise, adequate sleep, and a healthy diet can also help reduce stress and improve overall skin health.

By understanding the link between stress and eczema, and taking steps to manage stress effectively, you can help reduce flare-ups and improve the overall health of your skin. Remember, healing eczema is not just about treating the symptoms, but also addressing the underlying causes, including stress. With the right tools and strategies, you can take control of your eczema and achieve clear, healthy skin.

Stress-Relief Techniques for Eczema Sufferers

If you are one of the many people suffering from eczema, you know how stressful and frustrating it can be to deal with the constant itching, redness, and discomfort that comes with this skin condition. Stress is a known trigger for eczema flare-ups, so finding effective stress-relief techniques is essential for managing your symptoms and improving your overall well-being.

There are several stress-relief techniques that can help eczema sufferers find relief and improve their skin health. One of the most effective ways to reduce stress is through mindfulness and relaxation techniques such as deep breathing, meditation, and yoga. These practices can help calm your mind and body, reducing the release of stress hormones that can exacerbate eczema symptoms.

Exercise is another great way to relieve stress and improve your skin health. Physical activity releases endorphins, which are natural mood-boosting chemicals that can help reduce stress and anxiety. Regular exercise can also improve circulation, which is important for healing eczema-prone skin.

In addition to mindfulness, relaxation, and exercise, it's important to find healthy ways to cope with stress and manage your emotions. This may include talking to a therapist or counselor, practicing self-care activities such as taking a warm bath or reading a good book, or engaging in hobbies that bring you joy and relaxation.

By incorporating stress-relief techniques into your daily routine, you can help alleviate the symptoms of eczema and improve your overall quality of life. Remember to be patient and consistent with these practices, as it may take time to see results. With dedication and perseverance, you can find relief from eczema and enjoy clearer, healthier skin.

Mindfulness and Meditation for Eczema Relief

In the journey to healing eczema, it's important to not only focus on the physical aspects of the condition but also address the mental and emotional components that can exacerbate symptoms. Mindfulness and meditation are powerful tools that can help individuals cope with the stress and anxiety often associated with eczema, ultimately leading to relief and improved skin health.

Practicing mindfulness involves being fully present in the moment, without judgment or attachment to thoughts or emotions. This can help individuals with eczema manage their stress levels and prevent flare-ups triggered by anxiety or negative emotions. By cultivating a sense of calm and awareness, mindfulness can promote relaxation and reduce inflammation in the body, which can in turn improve skin condition.

Meditation, on the other hand, is a practice that involves focusing the mind on a particular object, thought, or activity to achieve mental clarity and emotional stability. For individuals with eczema, meditation can be a powerful tool for managing itching, pain, and discomfort associated with the condition. By redirecting attention away from the physical sensations of eczema and towards a peaceful state of mind, meditation can help individuals find relief and reduce the impact of eczema on their daily lives.

Incorporating mindfulness and meditation practices into a daily routine can have profound effects on overall well-being and skin health. By taking the time to connect with oneself and cultivate a sense of inner peace, individuals with eczema can experience relief from symptoms and a greater sense of control over their condition. Remember, healing eczema is not just about treating the skin—it's about nurturing the mind and body as a whole.

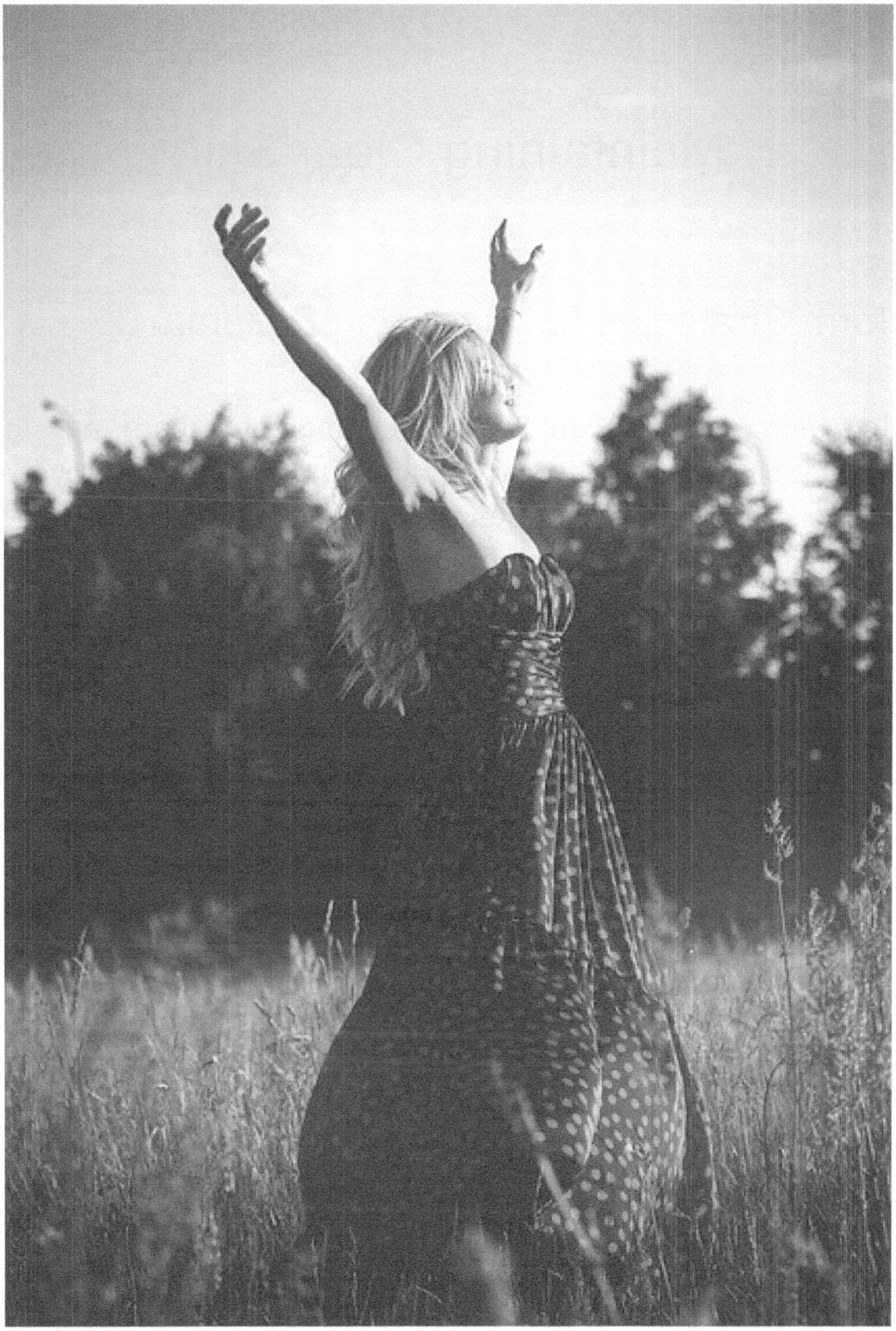

Chapter 7

Maintaining Clear Skin

Long-Term Strategies for Managing Eczema

Living with eczema can be challenging, but there are long-term strategies that can help you manage your symptoms and improve your skin health. By incorporating these strategies into your daily routine, you can take control of your eczema and experience clearer, healthier skin.

One of the most important long-term strategies for managing eczema is to establish a consistent skincare routine. This includes using gentle, fragrance-free products that are designed for sensitive skin. Moisturizing regularly can also help to keep your skin hydrated and reduce the risk of flare-ups.

In addition to skincare, it's important to pay attention to your diet and lifestyle. Some foods and environmental factors can trigger eczema flare-ups, so it's important to identify and avoid these triggers. Stress can also exacerbate eczema symptoms, so finding ways to manage and reduce stress in your life can be beneficial.

Another long-term strategy for managing eczema is to work closely with a healthcare provider. Your doctor can help you develop a treatment plan that is tailored to your specific needs and can recommend medications or other therapies that may help to control your symptoms.

Overall, managing eczema requires a holistic approach that addresses both the physical and emotional aspects of the condition. By incorporating these long-term strategies into your daily routine, you can take control of your eczema and experience clearer, healthier skin.

Preventing Eczema Flare-ups

Eczema flare-ups can be frustrating and uncomfortable, but there are steps you can take to prevent them and keep your skin clear and healthy. In this subchapter, we will discuss some effective strategies for preventing eczema flare-ups and maintaining clear skin.

One of the most important things you can do to prevent eczema flare-ups is to keep your skin moisturized. Dry skin is a common trigger for eczema, so using a gentle, fragrance-free moisturizer regularly can help keep your skin hydrated and prevent flare-ups.

In addition to keeping your skin moisturized, it is also important to avoid potential triggers that can exacerbate your eczema. Common triggers include harsh soaps, hot water, and certain fabrics like wool. By being mindful of these triggers and making small changes to your daily routine, you can help prevent flare-ups and keep your skin clear.

Another important aspect of preventing eczema flare-ups is managing stress. Stress can have a significant impact on your skin and may trigger flare-ups in some individuals. Finding healthy ways to manage stress, such as practicing yoga or meditation, can help reduce the likelihood of flare-ups and keep your skin looking its best.

Finally, it is important to pay attention to your diet and how it may be affecting your eczema. Some individuals find that certain foods can trigger flare-ups, so keeping a food diary and monitoring your symptoms can help you identify and avoid potential triggers.

By following these tips and being proactive about preventing eczema flare-ups, you can help keep your skin clear and healthy and enjoy a better quality of life. Remember, everyone's eczema triggers are different, so it may take some trial and error to find what works best for you.

Celebrating Your Eczema-Free Skin

After months or even years of dealing with the painful and frustrating symptoms of eczema, finally achieving clear, healthy skin is a moment worth celebrating. In this subchapter, we will explore ways to celebrate your eczema-free skin and embrace the new chapter of your life without the burden of constant flare-ups and itching.

One way to celebrate your eczema-free skin is by treating yourself to a spa day or pampering session. Indulge in a soothing bath with skin-nourishing oils and creams, or book a massage to relax and rejuvenate your body. Taking care of your skin is essential even after your eczema has cleared up, so continue to prioritize self-care and treat yourself to luxurious skincare products that will keep your skin healthy and glowing.

Another way to celebrate your newfound freedom from eczema is by sharing your journey with others. By opening up about your struggles and triumphs, you can inspire and encourage those who are still battling with eczema. Consider starting a blog or social media account to document your skincare routine, favorite products, and tips for managing eczema. Your story could make a difference in someone else's life and give them hope for their own healing journey.

Lastly, don't forget to thank yourself for all the hard work and dedication you put into healing your eczema. Celebrate your resilience and determination to overcome this challenging skin condition. Treat yourself to a special gift or plan a fun outing to commemorate this important milestone in your life.

Remember, achieving eczema-free skin is a significant accomplishment, and you deserve to celebrate every step of your healing journey. Embrace your new skin and enjoy the freedom that comes with being eczema-free.

Author Notes & Acknowledgments

First and foremost, I would like to express my deepest gratitude to the people who inspired and supported me throughout the journey of writing this book. This project would not have been possible without their unwavering belief in me and their invaluable contributions.

To my wife, thank you for your constant encouragement and understanding. Your love and support have been my anchor during the challenging times of researching and writing this book. Your belief in my ability to make a difference in people's lives has been my driving force.

I would also like to disclose that this book contains some renewed artificial intelligence-generated content. I really appreciate very recent technological innovation by outstanding scientists and of course our reader's understanding.

Lastly, I want to express my deepest gratitude to the readers of this book. I sincerely hope the strategies and methods outlined within these pages will provide you with the knowledge and tools needed to truly make your life much better. Your commitment to seeking any good solutions and willingness to explore multiple methods is commendable.

Author Bio

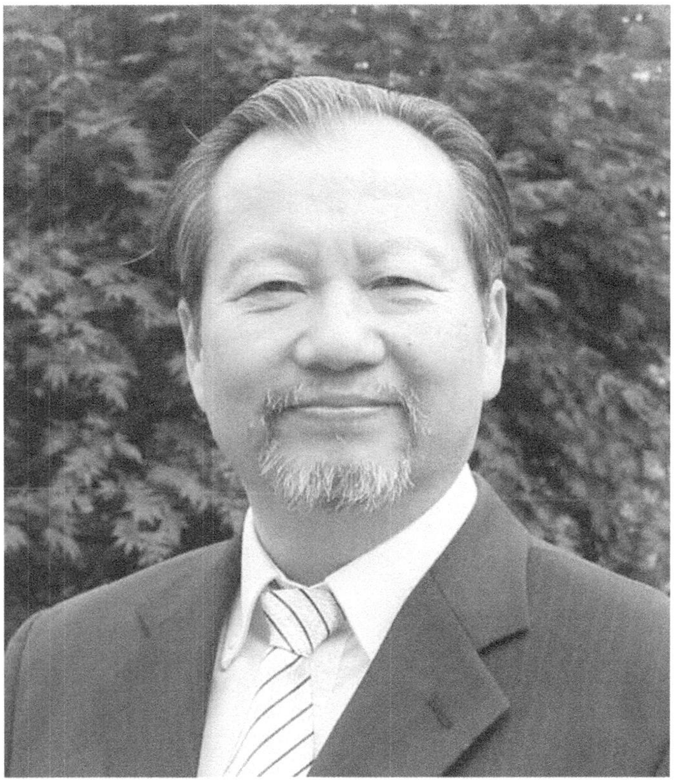

Johnson Wu earned his MD in 1982. With over 40 years of clinical experience, he has worked in hospitals in Zhejiang and Shanghai, China, as well as the Royal Marsden Hospital in London, UK.

Upon the recommendation of Sir Aaron Klug, the president of The Royal Society and a Nobel Prize winner in Chemistry, Dr. Wu was honorably awarded a British Royal Society Fellowship. He has published medical books and articles in seven countries and currently practices medicine in Canada.

Made in United States
Cleveland, OH
04 November 2026

47647244R00024